Khouloud Rmili
Iyadh Ghorbel
Khalil Ennouri

Regenerative therapy in the healing of acute burns

Khouloud Rmili
Iyadh Ghorbel
Khalil Ennouri

Regenerative therapy in the healing of acute burns

Analysis of innovative approaches to regenerative therapy and their clinical impact

ScienciaScripts

Imprint

Cover image: www.ingimage.com

This book is a translation from the original published under ISBN 978-613-9-52087-9.

Publisher:
Sciencia Scripts
is a trademark of
Dodo Books Indian Ocean Ltd. and OmniScriptum S.R.L publishing group

120 High Road, East Finchley, London, N2 9ED, United Kingdom
Str. Armeneasca 28/1, office 1, Chisinau MD-2012, Republic of Moldova, Europe
Managing Directors: Ieva Konstantinova, Victoria Ursu
info@omniscriptum.com

Printed at: see last page
ISBN: 978-620-8-57479-6

CONTENTS

INTRODUCTION

Burns are a major public health problem, causing around 180,000 deaths a year according to the WHO. They have considerable physical, psychological and financial repercussions for the victims and their families, leading to intense pain, disfiguring scars and organ dysfunction. These injuries are often accompanied by stigmatisation and rejection, which seriously affects patients' quality of life(1)

Traditional healing methods, such as wound healing and early excision-grafting, have long been the mainstays of burn treatment. Controlled wound healing, considered to be the first line of treatment for loss of skin substance, is based on the spontaneous healing process, without the use of sutures. It is based on the three phases of natural healing: detersion, budding and epithelialisation, with the aim of creating an environment conducive to healing. However, this approach can be compromised by factors such as infection and insufficient vascularisation(2)

In response to these limitations, early excision-grafting of burned areas, introduced in 1970 by Zora Janzekovic in Yugoslavia, has emerged as an effective technique. It is recommended for third-degree burns and, more frequently, for deep second-degree burns. In these cases, the affected tissues have little or no capacity to heal due to the almost total destruction of the epidermal cells. What's more, the necrosis of burned tissue leads to the release of toxins, increasing the risk of infection. It is therefore crucial, when the patient's general condition allows it, to excise the necrotic areas as soon as possible, ideally within the first five days. This helps to prevent infectious and toxic complications, while minimising the inflammatory reaction, malnutrition and skin retractions. Subsequently, the application of a skin graft to the debrided area promotes tissue regeneration by providing healthy cells and improving vascularisation. In addition, starting the excision and grafting protocol quickly helps to reduce the pain associated with prolonged dressings and shortens the length of hospital stay . (3)

However, although this method is favoured for its ability to accelerate healing, it does carry risks. Complications can arise, such as graft rejection, as well as post-operative problems such as bleeding or infection. In addition, although the main aim is to improve the aesthetics of healing, there is always a risk of hypertrophic or keloid scarring, which can compromise the final result . (4)

In recent years, the rapidly expanding field of regenerative therapy has opened up a new perspective on the management of acute burns. This innovative field combines advances in cell biology, bioengineering and gene therapy to develop treatments capable of regenerating damaged tissue, thereby promoting faster and more effective healing(5) . Thanks to their ability to differentiate into different cell types, stem cells make it possible to design personalised treatments tailored to the specific needs of each patient. With this in mind, the use of growth factors, biological matrices and cell therapies offers real hope of improving the quality of life of burn victims. However, despite the promising potential of regenerative therapy, its integration into clinical practice is controversial due to variations in results, the associated technical and ethical challenges, the lack of precise indications and its high cost, requiring rational and considered use.

In less developed countries, and Tunisia in particular, there are a number of problems associated with the treatment of burns. Firstly, the high cost of treatment and resources, combined with a lack of adequate funding, restricts access to care for a large proportion of the population. In addition, the prolonged healing time often requires long hospital stays, which can be difficult both psychologically and financially for families. Preventing post-operative complications also requires intensive care, but the capacity of care units is often limited, which further complicates management. These issues underline the need to improve healthcare infrastructures and increase the resources available to better meet the needs of burn victims in this country.

This is why we have chosen to carry out this systematic review, aimed at analysing recent studies on the application of regenerative therapy in the healing of acute burns. This review will summarise emerging technological innovations, assess their reliability and safety, and highlight their benefits. It will also address the challenges and future prospects of these revolutionary therapeutic approaches.

MATERIALS AND METHODS

1. Type of study

This study takes the form of a systematic review, based on an in-depth search of relevant databases, covering the publication period from 2015 to 2024. It provides a descriptive summary of the results of the selected studies, while adopting an analytical perspective to draw meaningful conclusions.

2. Inclusion

Studies were included if they met the following criteria:

- ➢ Randomised clinical trials investigating the use of regenerative therapies in the treatment of acute burns.
- ➢ Publications available in English or French, published between 2015 and 2024
- ➢ Studies of adult or paediatric populations with acute burns, whether or not surgery is required
- ➢ Use of regenerative medicine approaches, alone or in combination with conventional treatments such as skin grafts, to treat acute burns

3. Exclusion criteria

Studies were excluded if they met the following criteria:

- ➢ They focused on wound types other than acute burns, such as chronic burns, pressure sores or diabetic wounds, or they dealt with non-regenerative therapies.
- ➢ Non-randomised studies, preclinical or animal studies, case reports and theses.
- ➢ Articles for which access to the full text could not be obtained

4. Data sources and research strategy

4.1. Data sources

An exhaustive search was carried out in the following databases: "Medline" (via "PubMed"), "Elsevier" (via "Science Direct"), and "ResearchGate". These platforms were selected for their broad coverage of scientific publications in the fields of medicine and life sciences.

4.2. Research strategy

- The search was carried out using specific combinations of keywords and MeSH terms, such as: "Regenerative medicine", "Burns", "Wound healing", "Skin grafting", "Tissue engineering", "Stem cells", "Gene therapy", "Scar management", "Burn injuries", "growth factors", "skin regeneration", "acute burns", "clinical trials", and their French equivalents.
- The search strategy involved the use of Boolean operators (AND, OR) to combine these terms. Filters were applied to restrict results to studies published within the last ten years, to ensure inclusion of the most recent data.

5. Selection of studies

Initially, articles from the three databases were assessed on the basis of their title and abstract to determine their relevance. The articles deemed eligible were then examined in their entirety to check compliance with the inclusion criteria.

6. Data extraction and synthesis

- Relevant data were extracted using a standardised form. Information collected included study characteristics (author, year, type of study), participant characteristics (age, sex, type and severity of burns), interventions (type of regenerative therapy) and outcomes measured (time to healing, scar quality, pain, complications). Given the heterogeneity of the included studies, a narrative synthesis was adopted.

- The data collected was structured and presented in the form of tables and figures to facilitate comparison between studies. An in-depth discussion of the results was carried out to highlight recent advances, the limitations of current studies and the potential clinical implications of regenerative therapies.

7. Ethical considerations

All studies included in this review were examined to ensure that they had obtained approval from a local ethics committee and that informed consent had been obtained from participants. The ethical implications of using regenerative therapies to treat burns were considered, assessing the potential risks and benefits to patients. Particular attention was paid to protecting the rights and welfare of participants, especially with regard to experimental interventions and innovative therapeutic approaches.

➯ Definitions

❖ **Graft uptake** was the percentage of the graft that was vital and showed good adherence to the wound bed . (6)

❖ **Epithelialization** has been defined as the percentage of wound closure by a skin graft or outgrowth from the graft or wound edges . (6)

❖ **The Visual Analogue Thermometer (TVA)** a tool designed to measure pain in patients with burns. Adapted from the Visual Analogue Scale (VAS), the TVA uses a linear scale from 0 to 10 to quantify pain, where 0 means no pain and 10 represents the most intense pain possible. Patients indicate their level of pain by placing a marker on this scale, providing a subjective but quantifiable assessment. This tool is useful for detecting subtle variations in pain and adjusting therapeutic interventions accordingly(7)

❖ **The Patient and Observer Scar Assessment Scale (POSAS)** consists of two parts: assessment by the patient and assessment by the observer. The observer assessment includes six criteria: vascularisation, pigmentation, thickness, relief, malleability and general impression. The patient's assessment takes into account pain, itching, colour, rigidity, thickness and irregularity of the surface. Each criterion is scored on a scale from 1 to 10, and average scores are calculated for the two components . (8)

❖ **The DermaSpectrometer (Cortex Technology, Hadsund, Denmark)** is a validated instrument used to assess the colour and pigmentation of scars. It measures erythema (redness) and pigmentation (melanin) using a narrow-band reflectometer, providing an accurate and objective assessment of the colorimetric characteristics of scars . (9)

❖ **The Cutometer (Courage & Khazaka GmbH, Cologne, Germany)** is a device used to measure the elasticity of scars. It quantifies the vertical deformation of the skin in millimetres when it is sucked by controlled suction through a circular opening. The results are then expressed as a ratio to the values for normal skin, providing an accurate assessment of skin elasticity(10)

❖ **Nanofat** is a form of autologous fat obtained from lipoaspirate, transformed into a fluid, whitish product by a process of transfer between small syringes, usually around 30 times. This preparation is then applied in a thin layer to wounds, covered with Vaseline gauze and a sterile dressing, to promote healing and tissue regeneration.

RESULTS

A search of the three databases PubMed, Science Direct and ResearchGate identified 50 publications with relevant descriptors, covering a particularly fruitful publication period from 2015 to 2024. After a rigorous selection process based on a review of titles and abstracts, 42 publications were excluded for not meeting the selection criteria, notably because of their focus on subjects such as chronic burns, pressure sores, diabetic wounds, non-regenerative therapies, as well as non-randomised studies, preclinical or animal research, case reports, theses, or those without access to the full text. Following a full reading of the remaining 10 articles and application of the analysis criteria, a further 4 publications were excluded, resulting in a final selection of 4 relevant articles, all of which were randomised clinical trials (**Figure 1**). The main results of these trials are summarised **in Table I**.

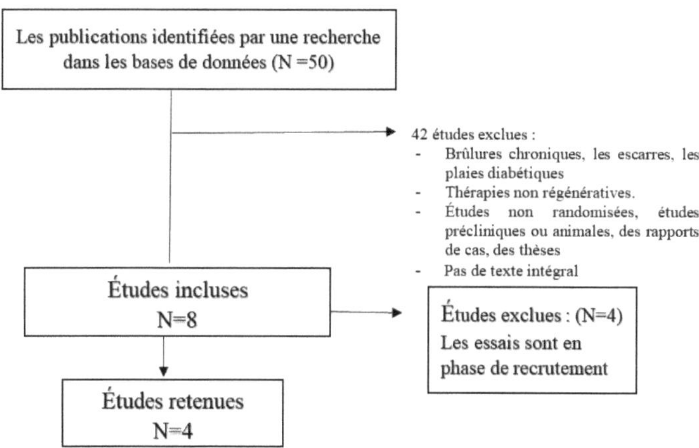

Figure 1 : Processus de sélection

Table I: Summary of the results of clinical trials on the healing of acute burns

	title	Authors, year of publication and countries	Main results
Article 1	The application of platelet-rich plasma in the treatment of deep dermal burns: A randomized, double-blind, intra- patient controlled study	Roos E et al The Netherlands 2016	the addition of PRP to the treatment of burns has not improved graft uptake or epithelialisation of deep dermal burns, nor has it been shown to improve scar quality.
Article 2	Efficacy of Lyophilised Platelet-Rich Plasma Powder on Healing Rate in Patients With Deep Second Degree Burn Injury: A Prospective Double-Blind Randomized Clinical Trial	Chi-Yung Yeung et al Taiwan, Republic of China 2017	Quadruple application of freeze-dried PRP significantly improves the healing of deep second-degree burns after three weeks.
Article 3	New procedure: Do sequential skin cell grafts heal third-degree burns? Comparative study of 517 patients	Sabeh G et al Lebanon	Sequential skin grafts have shown promising results for deep second-degree burns and could also benefit third-degree burns, particularly with the addition of PRP and cryoprecipitated plasma.
Article 4	Effect of autologous fat transfer in acute burn wound management: A randomized controlled study	Ahmed M. Abouzaid et al Egypt 2021	Autologous fat grafting has shown significant clinical benefits, including a reduction in the length of hospitalisation, the need for additional surgery and contractures. It also reduces the need for skin grafts and improves the quality of scars compared with conventional treatments.

We reviewed four randomised clinical trials of regenerative

therapy approaches for the treatment of acute burns. Each study has distinct objectives, methodologies and outcomes. The research focuses on platelet-rich plasma (PRP), lyophilised PRP (LRP), sequential skin cell transplantation (SSCT) and autologous fat transfer.

A randomised, double-blind, intra-patient controlled trial was conducted at the Dutch Burn Center of the Red Cross Hospital in Beverwijk, the Netherlands. Its aim was to test the hypothesis that PRP containing autologous leukocytes improves the healing of acute burns and the quality of scars. The effect of PRP was assessed on the rate of graft uptake, epithelialisation of deep dermal burns, and scar quality at 3, 6 and 12 months post-surgery.

Between June 2010 and January 2014, a total of 52 patients aged 18 years and older (mean age 51.2 ± 18.6 years, with a sex ratio of 1.48) with deep dermal burns covering at least 2% of total body surface area (mean burned body surface area 51.6 ± 14.5%) and requiring thin skin grafting were included. Two comparable wound areas were randomly assigned to PRP or control treatment. PRP was applied prior to grafting, followed by a non-adhesive dressing left in place for 5-7 days.

The study, conducted in China in 2017, examined the effect of freeze-dried PRP (PRPL) on the healing of deep second-degree burns covering between 10% and 48% of the total body surface area, focusing on fibroblast proliferation and the frequency of treatment application. PRPL was applied daily for four days to the burns (quadruple application of PRPL demonstrated significant stimulation of fibroblast proliferation, considered crucial for the initial phase of healing), with monitoring of the healing process. Patients with a history of cancer, allergies or transfusion reactions were excluded from the study. The study included 27 patients divided into two groups: a PRPL group (n=15) and a control group (n=12). PRPL, at a concentration of 1.0 × 10^7 platelets/cm² according to wound size, was uniformly applied. Endpoints included percentage wound closure and bacterial clearance rate after 2 and 3 weeks of treatment.

Among the 27 patients included, there were 18 men and 9 women, with a mean age of 45.27 ± 15.82 years in the PRPL group and 46.00 ± 14.03 years in the control group ($p=0.45$). The sex ratio was 3 in the control group and 1.5 in the PRPL group. With regard to wound location, the control group had 7 cases on the upper limbs and 5 on the lower limbs, while the PRPL group had 7 cases on the upper limbs and 8 on the lower limbs. The mean surface area of the burns was 75.63 ± 50.72 cm² for the control group and 99.73 ± 70.17 cm² for the PRPL group ($p=0.16$).

The collaborative study conducted by the Burnology Department and the Cellular Engineering Laboratory at Peace Hospital in Bahsas, Lebanon, was carried out to evaluate the efficacy of GSCCs as an alternative to tissue grafts to treat deep electrical burns. Between February 2012 and June 2016, 478 patients were included in the study. Of the 478 patients included in the study, 206 were infants, 109 were children aged between 3 and 13 years, and 202 were adults. Infants were studied separately due to their distinct burn characteristics and outcome measures. Children and adults were grouped together to limit the complexity of subgroups.

It has been shown that burns observed in children and adults have similar characteristics in terms of the causal agent, the areas affected and the surface and depth of the burns.

In infants, burns were mainly caused by hot liquids (90% of cases vs. 40% in children and adults, $p < 0.0001$), with more frequent involvement of the trunk (65% vs. 43%, $p < 0.0001$) and less frequent involvement of the hands (28% vs. 47%, $p < 0.005$). All patients had at least deep second-degree burns, while 29% of infants and 33% of children/adults had third-degree burns. The mean burned area was 22% in infants and 28.5% in children/adults ($p<0.0001$).

The patients were divided into four groups:

- **Group 1 (Control)**: 97 patients (20%), including 26 infants and 71 children/adults, who refused GSCC and were treated by debridement, with or without tissue grafting.
- **Group 2 (GSCC)**: 264 patients (55%), including 148 children/adults and 116 infants, treated with GSCC between February 2012 and April 2015.
- **Group 3 (GSCC+)**: 77 patients (16%), including 47 children/adults and 30 infants, treated with GSCC with PRP for the first three procedures and plasma cryoprecipitate (CP) for the subsequent ones, from April 2015.
- **Group 4 (GSCC+/-)**: 40 patients (8%), including 17 infants and 23 children/adults, treated with two comparable zones: one with GSCC alone and the other with GSCC combined with PRP and CP.

The clinical study, conducted from March 2019 to March 2020 in the burns unit of Aboqir General Hospital in Alexandria, Egypt, aimed to evaluate the effect of autologous fat transfer to treat acute burns. It included one hundred patients, aged between 14 and 45 years, of any sex, in stable general condition, with superficial or deep dermal burns covering between 10% and 25% of the total body surface area. Exclusion criteria included burns involving deep layers (fat, fascia, muscle, bone), inhalation burns, or burns affecting the genital, perineal and perianal organs. Patients with co-morbidities influencing healing or suitability for anaesthesia, such as diabetes, vascular, immunological, renal, hepatic or cardiac disease, or stroke, were also excluded.

Patients were divided into two groups: group A (50 patients) received an injection of autologous fat graft followed by a dressing with nanofat, while group B (50 patients) was treated with successive conventional dressings using topical agents such as silver sulphadiazine and mafenide. Baseline patient characteristics and demographics (age, gender, percentage of body surface area burned, burn type and depth, and wound site) were comparable between the two groups, with no significant differences (**Table II**).

Table II: Comparison between the two groups studied according to various parameters

	Cases (n = 50)	Control (n = 50)	Test of Sig.	p
Number of times to OR for each case				
Mean ± SD	1.3 ± 0.6	2 ± 1.4	U= 807.0*	< 0.001*
Median (Min. – Max.)	1(1 – 3)	2(1 – 6)		
Opioid analgesia use				
None given	39(78%)	1(2%)	χ^2 = 60.167*	< 0.001*
Prescribed	11(22%)	49(98%)		
Frequency of dressing change				
Daily	5(10%)	50(100%)	χ^2 = 81.818*	< 0.001*
Day after another	15(30%)	0(0%)		
Every 2 days	30(60%)	0(0%)		
Use of Chemical Topical agents				
No Topical medication	45(90%)	0(0%)	χ^2 = 81.818*	< 0.001*
Topical medication	5(10%)	50(100%)		
Skin grafting				
No skin graft	40(80%)	26(52%)	χ^2 = 8.734*	0.003*
Skin graft	10(20%)	24(48%)		
Frequency of visits in the outpatient clinic				
Mean ± SD.	2 ± 1.8	10 ± 2.4	U= 10.0*	< 0.001*
Median (Min. – Max.)	2(0 – 5)	10(5 – 14)		
Re-admission				
No	40(80%)	31(62%)	χ^2 = 3.934*	0.047*
Yes	10(20%)	19(38%)		
Hospital stay				
Mean ± SD.	12.6 ± 3.8	19.2 ± 4.2	t = 8.265*	< 0.001*
Median (Min. – Max.)	13.5(1 – 20)	19(10 – 30)		
Scar				
Scar Texture				
Smooth texture	40(80%)	16(32%)	χ^2 = 23.377*	< 0.001*
Rough Texture	10(20%)	34(68%)		
Surface level to surrounding				
Normal	45(90%)	14(28%)	χ^2 = 39.727*	< 0.001*
Hyper trophic	5(10%)	36(72%)		
Hyper pigmented				
Normal	40(80%)	8(16%)	χ^2 = 41.026*	< 0.001*
Colored	10(20%)	42(84%)		
Hypo pigmented				
Normal	45(90%)	10(20%)	χ^2 = 49.495*	< 0.001*
Colored	5(10%)	40(80%)		
Contractures				
No	45(90%)	32(64%)	χ^2 = 9.543*	0.002*
Yes	5(10%)	18(36%)		

χ2: Chi square test. t: Student t-test. U: Mann Whitney test. p: p-value for comparing between the studied groups. *: Statistically significant at $p \leq 0.05$.

Effects of Regenerative Therapy on the Healing Process

According to the study by Roos E et al, no statistically significant difference was observed in mean graft take and epithelialization rates between PRP-treated and control areas at day 5-7 (Mann-Whitney test; p=0.23 and p=0.1, respectively). However, when classified as 'equal, better or worse', PRP-treated areas were significantly more likely to have 'equal or better' graft take and epithelialization rates than control areas (chi-square test; p=0.007 for graft take and p=0.02 for epithelialization).

In addition, analyses showed that, for patients operated on early (within 7 days of the burn, n=11), uptake rates were significantly higher in the PRP group compared with standard care, with a mean difference of 12.7% (t-test, p=0.036; 95% CI: 1.0-24.3). Similarly, surgery within 7 days was also a significant predictor of better epithelialisation rates, with a mean difference of 9.3% (t-test, p=0.033; 95% CI: 0.8-17.8). No differences were observed between patients operated on within 7 days and those operated on after 7 days in terms of age, percentage of body surface burnt, platelet count or gender.

Chi-Yung Yeung et al. reported that in the control group, the initial wound surface area was 25.49 cm². After two weeks, this surface area had decreased to 23.79 cm², representing a healing rate of 6.67%. After three weeks, the wound area had decreased to 4.34 cm², corresponding to a healing rate of 86.40%. However, in the PRPL group, the initial wound area was 84.36 cm². By week 2, this had reduced to 23.96 cm², representing 71.59% healing. At week 3, the surface area was 0.63 cm², corresponding to 99.24% of total healing.

Two weeks after the start of treatment, mean wound closure rates were 65.61 ± 32.3% in the control group and 75.64 ± 20.38% in the PRPL group, with no statistically significant difference between the two groups. However, after three weeks, the closure rate was 85.3 ± 15.13% in the control group versus 92.99 ± 6.24% in the PRPL group, indicating a significant difference ($p < 0.05$).

Representative photographs of the cases are shown in **Figure 2** :

Typical deep second degree burns on the plantar region of the feet after debridement and cleansing were studied. The percentage of wound closure after application of PRPL or placebo solution at weeks

2 and 3 was measured. (The area of the wounds after application of the PRPL/placebo solution is surrounded by a white line).

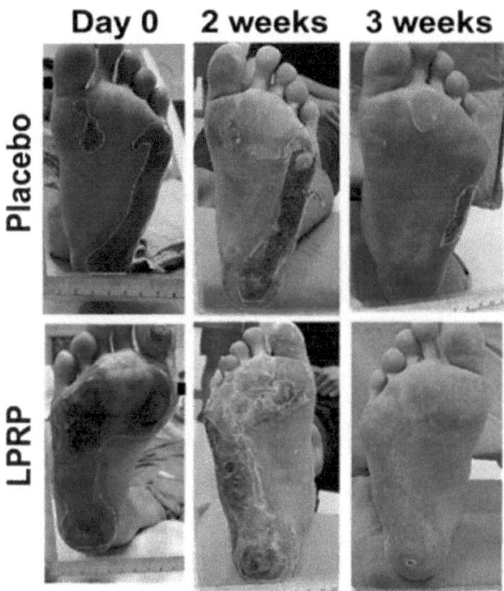

Figure 2: Comparison of the clinical presentation of the PRPL group and the control group at days 0, 2 and 3 weeks.

In the study by Sabeh G et al, second degree burns treated with GSCC healed without grafting in 6 to 8 days (6 days with PRP and CP, 8 days without PRP and CP). In the control group, spontaneous healing took 25 days, and healing with tissue grafting took 20 days. For third-degree burns, healing took 47 days with the addition of PRP and CP and 55 days with GSCC alone (**Figure 3**).

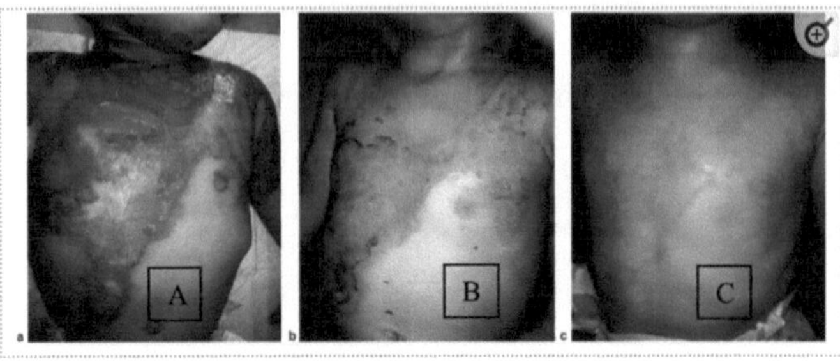

**Figure 3: 2nd degree burn A- before treatment, B- appearance on day 4 of GSCC,
C- Epidermisation at D8**

Research conducted by Ahmed M. Abouzaid et al. showed that group A had a significant reduction in the total number of days spent in hospital, with an average of 12.6 ± 3.8 days compared with 19.2 ± 4.2 days for the control group ($p < 0.001$). In addition, group A required fewer trips to the operating theatre, with an average of 1.3 ± 0.6 compared with 2 ± 1.4 ($p < 0.001$), and needed fewer additional skin grafts (20% compared with 48%, $p = 0.003$). Finally, the number of outpatient consultations after discharge was also reduced in group A, with a mean of 2 ± 1.8 compared with 10 ± 2.4 for the control group ($p < 0.001$).

Importantly, less nanofat was used for topical dressings in the group treated with autologous fat, suggesting a reduction in wound size and improved wound healing (**Figure 4**).

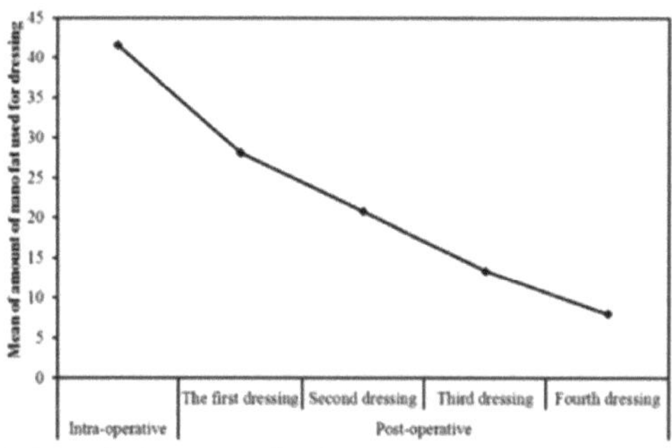

Figure 4: Descriptive analysis of cases according to the quantity of nanogrease applied for the coating

Regenerative therapy and its impact on pain

In the study by Roos E et al, there was no significant difference in mean pain and itch scores, assessed using the visual analogue thermometer, between areas treated with PRP and those without. In contrast, patients treated with autologous fat generally underwent a single surgical procedure and did not require dressings under anaesthesia. This indicates significantly less pain compared with patients in the control group, who had to undergo up to six procedures and dressings under anaesthetic.

Regenerative therapy and complications

For patients treated with PRP, no significant difference was found in bacterial colonisation rates between the two groups. No serious adverse events, such as allergic reactions, sepsis or death, were reported. However, eight patients (16%) required re-operation, with a higher incidence in those operated on within seven days of the burn (Mann-Whitney test, $p = 0.011$). Although reoperation was more frequent in the PRP group, it was not associated with a higher percentage of burnt body surface or a larger mesh size (Mann-Whitney test, $p = 0.28$ and $p = 0.30$, respectively). Among cases requiring re-operation, areas treated with PRP were significantly smaller than those treated with standard methods (45% versus 58%, p = 0.049, Mann-Whitney test).

For freeze-dried PRP, the postoperative infection rate was 26.67% in the LRP group, compared with 33.33% in the control group. The p-values for preoperative and postoperative infections were 0.4427 and 0.3496 respectively, indicating that there was no significant difference between the two groups.

Regenerative therapy: effects on scar quality

For long-term results, scar quality was assessed on an outpatient basis at 3, 6 and 12 months after the procedure, using both objective and subjective measurement tools. At all three times, there were no significant differences between the areas treated with PRP and those receiving standard care in terms of POSAS scores, colour and pigmentation measured with the DermaSpectrometer, and skin elasticity assessed with the Cutometer. On the other hand, a significant improvement in scar texture was observed in patients who received autologous fat transfer. After 6 months, 80% of patients in Group A had smooth scars, compared with only 32% in the control group ($p<0.001$). Furthermore, 90% of patients in group A did not develop keloid or hypertrophic scars, whereas 28% of controls developed these types of scars ($p< 0.001$). Finally, only 10% of patients who received autologous fat grafting developed contractures, compared with 36% in the control group ($p<0.002$) (**Figure 5**).

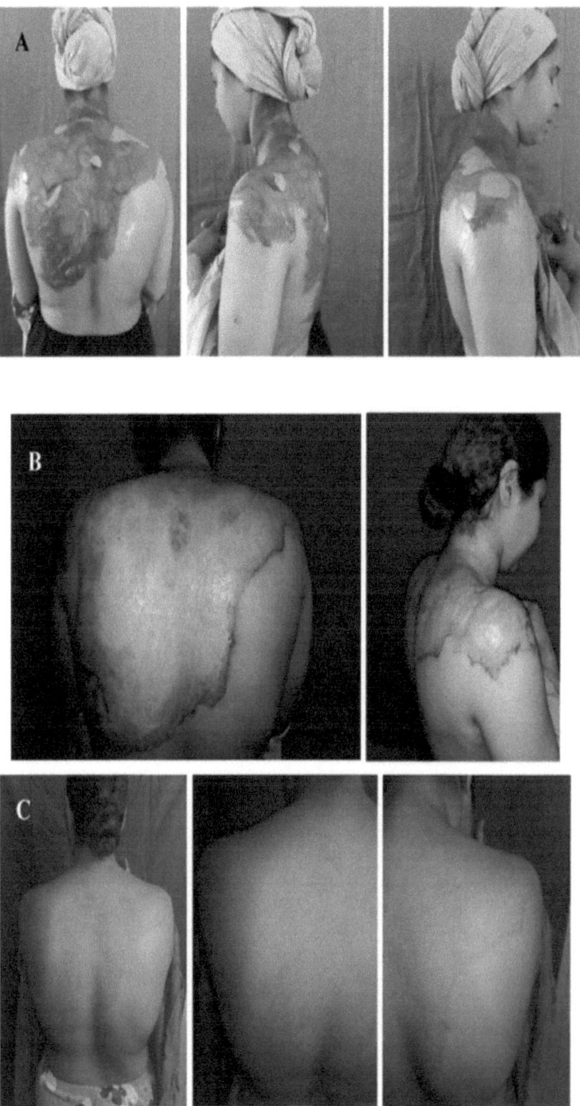

Figure 5: 24-year-old woman suffering from a scald burn with deep lesions in the dermis: (A) Pre-treatment with fat autograft and topical application of nanofat, (B) First week after treatment. (C) 6 months after treatment, note minimal colour change and absence of contractures.

Mortality

In the sequential skin cell transplant study, overall mortality was observed at 4.25%, with a total of 22 deaths, distributed as follows: 10 infants, 5 children and 7 adults. The average length of hospital stay was 15 days for infants, and 20 days for children and adults.

DISCUSSION

Platelet-rich plasma is a blood fraction that contains a concentration of platelets three to five times higher than that of whole blood, i.e. between 800,000 and 1,000,000 platelets/mm^3(11) . Used in various medical sectors such as bone regeneration, cosmetic surgery and the treatment of acute, chronic and diabetic wounds(12) , PRP was first applied in 1987 in a case of cardiac surgery in Italy . (13)

Its properties for clinical use are mainly linked to its viscosity, which acts as a biological glue, its haemostatic action and the numerous growth factors contained in the platelet granules, which are released into the surrounding environment during platelet aggregation. In fact, once activated, platelets release various growth factors, such as platelet-derived growth factor (PDGF), fibroblast growth factor (FGF), transforming growth factor b (TGF-b) and epidermal growth factor (EGF), vascular endothelial growth factor (VEGF) and insulin-like growth factor (IGF) , which are essential for wound healing by promoting chemotaxis, cell adhesion, mitogenesis, proliferation and angiogenesis(14,15) . Platelets also have antimicrobial and analgesic properties . (16,17)

There are several methods of preparing PRP, each varying in cost, composition (with or without leukocytes), and structure (fluid, gel, fibrin). It can also be activated in a variety of ways and can be prepared from autologous or allogeneic blood . (18)

Studies on PRP have mainly focused on healthy individuals, which poses specific challenges for its use in burn patients. In this population, physiological alterations and already activated platelets complicate the application of PRP. It is also impractical to draw blood prior to surgery to avoid prior platelet activation. In addition, the impact of burns on platelet quality and the hypercoagulable state of patients may influence the efficacy of PRP and determine the most appropriate time for its application . (19)

The literature recommends a platelet concentration of over 1000 x 10^3/mL in PRP(20) . According to the study by Roos et al, 73% of samples reached this level. However, sub-analyses showed that platelet concentration did not significantly affect outcomes, suggesting that platelet quality and content are also crucial. In addition, this double-blind randomised trial showed that the addition of PRP to the surgical treatment of deep burns did not significantly improve graft uptake and epithelialisation compared with wounds treated by surgery alone. However, minor benefits of PRP were observed in patients operated on early (7 days after the burn), including equal or higher rates of graft uptake and epithelialisation, as well as a reduction in the size of areas requiring re-operation . (21)

In terms of pain management, although PRP is known for its analgesic properties, the study by Roos et al. found no significant effect on pain or itching. This may be due to the inability to fully assess pain in some critically ill patients (intubation or severe burns)(21) . Also, no significant difference was observed with respect to bacterial colonisation or severe infections ,(21) calling into question the potential protective efficacy of leukocytes present in PRP, as mentioned in the literature.

Some researchers suggest that the leukocytes present in PRP could exacerbate inflammation, potentially detrimental to scar quality. Growth factors such as TGF-β1, TGF-β2, and PDGF, released by platelets and leukocytes in PRP, could prolong inflammation and lead to hypertrophic scars . (22)

Although the study by Roos et al. found no evidence of hypertrophic scarring associated with PRP(21) , no significant difference in scar quality was observed between burns treated with PRP and those treated using standard methods . (23)

Although liquid PRP is considered a reference treatment in several medical fields, its use in burns is limited due to technical difficulties such as the need for continuous agitation, a high risk of contamination, and a short shelf life .(24)

To overcome these challenges, a freeze-dried PRP powder has been introduced as an advanced solution. This freeze-drying process, which consists of dehydrating the PRP in a vacuum, combined with gamma-ray sterilisation, provides better thermal stability, with a reduced risk of contamination and an extended shelf life. Compared with liquid PRP, freeze-dried PRP simplifies administration, allows prolonged release of growth factors, and enhances its regenerative effects. In practical terms, it can be stored at room temperature at the nursing station and administered directly to the patient, making it easier and more convenient to use in clinics .(25,26)

For lyophilised PRP to be used effectively in wound healing, two critical factors need to be considered: concentration and frequency of application. It is essential to maintain a minimum concentration of 0.8 to

1 × 10^6 platelets/mL to ensure effective wound healing. In the study by Chi-Yung Yeung et al, each vial of freeze-dried PRP, when dissolved in 50 mL of sterile water and applied evenly over a 100 cm^2 area, achieved a concentration of 1.0 × 10^7 platelets/mL, which has been found to be effective in previous research . (18,24)

Standard clinical protocols generally recommend a single application of freeze-dried PRP. However, the study by Yeung CY et al. found that patients treated with freeze-dried PRP for the first four days had faster wound closure in three weeks compared to the control group(27) . In addition, a comparative study demonstrated that the daily application of freeze-dried PRP promoted faster wound healing than the use of silver sulphadiazine . (21,28)

There is growing interest in the application of PRP for the treatment of acute burns, but its clinical benefits remain controversial. The lack of significant results in some studies raises questions about its efficacy, particularly with regard to the quality of PRP, which may be impaired in burn patients due to premature activation or degradation of platelets. In addition, the concentration of platelets in PRP may be insufficient, especially in the case of extensive burns or low platelet counts, and the optimal level required to improve healing is not yet defined. The frequency with which PRP is applied could also influence its effectiveness. Some research, such as that by Picard et al, suggests that repeated applications may be required to achieve significant results . (29)

Variations in results observed in the literature may be due to differences in PRP products, preparation methods or to potentially limited efficacy of the PRP itself. A promising alternative is allogeneic PRP, which could offer advantages in terms of standardisation and availability, avoiding the need for blood collection in burn patients. However, this approach raises concerns about biocompatibility and the potential risks of transmitting infections or allergic reactions, similar to those observed with platelet transfusions. Although case reports have not revealed any major side effects, further studies are needed to fully assess the safety and efficacy of this method . (12,30)

Skin grafts, an ancient practice, have evolved significantly since they were first used in Antiquity. A major turning point came in 1869, when Reverdin introduced the "epidermal graft". Since then, grafting techniques have diversified to include half-thickness and whole skin grafts. These techniques, whether temporary (allo- and xenografts) or permanent (autografts), aim to accelerate epidermalisation, which is crucial to the survival and functional results of patients suffering from burns . (31,32)

Since the 1950s, cell therapy has taken a new step forward with the trypsinisation technique developed by A. and H. Moscona, enabling the separation and culture of skin cells(33) . Among recent innovations, Sequential Transplants of Skin Cells stand out as a notable advance. This method involves separating and implanting the three layers of skin from a small healthy sample in burned areas. Thanks to its autologous and physiological approach, GSCCs promote complete epidermisation and are showing promising results for deep second-degree burns, and potentially for third-degree burns traditionally treated with tissue grafts(34) . Indeed, results obtained by Sabeh G et al. show significant improvements with the sequential use of cell lines combined with PRP, CP, antioxidants and wound healing stimulants(34) . After seeding, stem cells interact with skin cells, releasing cytokines and growth factors that promote tissue regeneration. For second-degree burns, the application of juxtaposed epidermal cells and dermal cells accelerates epidermalisation(35,36) . For third-degree burns, it is essential to reconstruct the dermis with dermal and hypodermal cells before supplementing with epidermal and dermal cells for effective skin reconstitution . (37)

It is essential to stress that the best results in cell therapy are often obtained when combined with adjuvant treatments. Platelets play a key role in releasing cytokines and growth factors that stimulate wound healing and cell migration, and also have antimicrobial properties(38) . PRP, in particular, with its high platelet concentration, significantly reduces the healing time of second-degree burns(18) . In addition, CP, rich in albumin, immunoglobulins, fibrinogen and fibronectin, promotes cell adhesion and improves wound healing by regulating the interactions between the extracellular matrix and cells thanks to fibronectin(39) . Agents such as olive oil(40) , which is rich in antioxidants, and honey(41,42) , known for its antimicrobial and healing properties, also contribute to better burn healing. Vitamins also play a crucial role: vitamin C(43) is essential for collagen synthesis, vitamin K(44) helps prevent clotting disorders and vitamin A(45) promotes epithelial regeneration at the end of treatment. Finally, to maximise the effectiveness of grafting and cell therapy techniques, it is essential to ensure adequate nutrition (macro- and micronutrition) and appropriate pain management, which are crucial prerequisites for optimal healing . (46,47)

The autologous fat transfer technique, first described in 1893 by Franz Neuber, was designed to fill a cheek defect caused by tuberculosis of the maxilla, fat taken from a patient's arm(48) . Although this method was explored in the twentieth century for filling soft tissue, the results were often inconsistent. It was only after Sydney Coleman established a rigorous protocol for fat harvesting and injection that results became more reliable. Since then, fat grafting has grown in popularity and its clinical applications have diversified . (49)

With the advent of liposuction in the 1980s, interest in autologous fat grafting was revived. Today, it is widely recognised not only for its ability to restore volume, but also for its regenerative properties. The technique is valued for its ability to differentiate into various tissues, such as fat, bone, cartilage and muscle(50,51) . In fact, the stromal vascular fraction of fat, rich in multipotent stem cells, plays a crucial role in the regeneration of damaged tissue. These stem cells, mainly present in lipoaspirate taken from the lower abdomen and inner thighs, have angiogenic, immunomodulatory and anti-apoptotic properties. They therefore help to improve the survival and volume of fat grafts . (52,53)

Recent research has also shown that stem cells derived from adipose tissue can reduce the tension and thickness of scars, accelerate revascularisation and reduce the fibrosis associated with thermal burns. They promote healing by differentiating into fibroblasts and keratinocytes, while secreting growth factors (PDGF, EGF, TGF-b, FGF, HGF (hepatic growth factor)), anti-inflammatory cytokines and peptides such as leptin and adiponectin. This contributes to better tissue repair . (54,55)

The effectiveness of fat grafting in the treatment of burns is well documented, with numerous studies attesting to its positive impact on the healing and fibrosis of acute and sub-acute wounds. For example, research by Piccolo et al. has shown that fat grafting promotes healing of burns after three weeks or more, with no apparent progression of lesions, and helps to accelerate the healing process of vascular ulcers while reducing the risk of hypertrophic scarring(56) . These results are supported by the work of Abouzaid et al, who also observed a reduction in scar thickness and an improvement in the suppleness of healed skin(57) . In addition, cases reported by Klinger et al. in 2008 showed an improvement in scar quality in patients who had suffered facial burns after fat grafting . (58)

In terms of its effect on pain, studies by Fredman et al. have shown that the application of fat grafting to complex burn scars, often accompanied by neuropathic pain, leads to a significant improvement in patients' symptoms. Their study concludes that fat grafting is an effective approach to the management of difficult scars, providing not only significant pain relief but also an overall improvement in patients' quality of life. This method therefore offers a promising alternative for the treatment of complications associated with burns . (59)

However, it is important to emphasise that these studies have limitations that must be taken into account if the results are to be accurately interpreted

Firstly, a high drop-out rate in follow-up assessments is a significant limitation. This problem is probably attributable to the distance between patients and the hospital or national burns treatment centre. Such a high drop-out rate could lead to an underestimation of rare adverse events, although patients with severe wound healing problems are likely to have returned to the facility. This gap in follow-up may nevertheless influence long-term results, thereby skewing conclusions about the prolonged effects of treatment.

Secondly, the heterogeneity of the sample is an important factor in the variability of the results observed. The patient group represents a diverse clinical sample, illustrating the variety of cases treated. This diversity includes variations in the size of areas treated, skin graft expansion, timing of surgery and platelet count, which could explain the wide variability in results obtained.

Thirdly, although sequential skin cell grafts do not affect mortality, which is mainly influenced by early escharotomy, the time to healing of third-degree burns is longer with GSCCs compared with excision-graft techniques. This highlights the need to re-evaluate their use in these specific cases.

Fourthly, although the reassuring history of autologous fat transfer since the 19th century alleviates certain concerns, the potential risk of tumour transformation of the transplanted stem cells remains a limitation to be considered.

Finally, the study carried out at the burns unit of the Aboqir General Hospital in Alexandria, Egypt, has limitations due to the absence of double blinding, which means that neither the participants nor the researchers were blind to the treatment administered. This lack of double-blinding may introduce bias, as the participants' expectations and behaviours, as well as the researchers' observations, may be influenced by their knowledge of the treatment. As a result, the results could be partially affected by subjective factors rather than by effects strictly linked to the interventions studied. In addition, the relatively small sample size limits the generalisability of the conclusions, as a small sample may not adequately represent the total population, increasing the risk of statistical error and reducing the reliability of the results.

CONCLUSION

Regenerative therapy, notably through the use of Platelet Rich Plasma (PRP), freeze-dried PRP, sequential skin grafts and autologous fat grafting, represents a significant advance in the treatment of acute burns. The four randomised clinical trials reviewed in this brief provided varied perspectives on these approaches, revealing both successes and limitations.

Results on liquid PRP are heterogeneous. Some studies have shown significant benefits, such as improved clinical outcomes, faster healing and pain relief in the treatment of acute burns. However, other research has not shown significant benefits. This disparity may be explained by the variability of PRP preparation techniques, including platelet and growth factor concentrations, which differ between manufacturers. This highlights the importance of standardising PRP preparation and application protocols in order to optimise its efficacy and safety.

Freeze-dried PRP has proven its effectiveness in the treatment of deep second-degree burns by accelerating healing and reducing bacterial contamination. It offers a number of advantages over liquid PRP, including better thermal stability, longer shelf life and reduced risk of contamination. It is easy to store and administer in the clinic, making it even more practical. In addition, it allows a prolonged release of growth factors, enhancing its regenerative effects. However, more in-depth comparative studies are needed to assess its relative efficacy compared with liquid PRP.

Sequential skin grafts are emerging as a promising alternative, offering significant added value in the treatment of severe burns. They are showing encouraging results for deep second-degree burns and could also be beneficial for third-degree burns, particularly when combined with PRP and cryoprecipitated plasma. Sequential skin cell transplantation could thus complement other tissue grafting techniques and skin substitutes, proving particularly useful in situations where there is a shortage of skin or where therapeutic options are limited.

Autologous fat grafting has demonstrated significant clinical advantages over conventional methods. It reduces the length of hospital stay, the need for additional surgery and contractures. In addition, this technique reduces the need for skin grafts and improves the quality of scars compared with traditional treatments. These results highlight the importance of paying greater attention to this approach in future research and clinical practice.

In conclusion, although regenerative therapies offer promising prospects for the healing of acute burns, further research is needed to refine these approaches. Future studies should aim to improve the quality and standardisation of PRP products, compare liquid and freeze-dried forms of PRP, optimise application protocols, and further evaluate the benefits of sequential skin grafts and autologous fat grafts. These efforts will help to improve clinical outcomes and ensure better management of acute burns

BIBLIOGRAPHY

1. Mashadi-Abdollahi H, Sadeghi H, Maghsoudi, Ranjbar, Soudmand. Stress disorder and PTSD after burn injuries: a prospective study of predictors of PTSD at Sina Burn Center, Iran. Neuropsychiatr Dis Treat. July 2011;425.

2. Revol M, Servant JM. Directed wound healing. EMC - Tech Chir - Chir Plast Reconstr Esthét. Jan 2010;5(1):1-9.

3. Chaouat M, Zakine G, Mimoun M. Principles of local management: surgical treatments. Pathol Biol. June 2011;59(3):e57-61.

4. Lloyd ECO, Rodgers BC. Outpatient Burns: Prevention and Care. 2012;85(1).

5. Rowan MP, Cancio LC, Elster EA, Burmeister DM, Rose LF, Natesan S, et al. Burn wound healing and treatment: review and advancements. Crit Care. June 12, 2015;19:243.

6. Bloemen MCT, Boekema BKHL, Vlig M, Van Zuijlen PPM, Middelkoop E. Digital image analysis versus clinical assessment of wound epithelialization: A validation study. Burns. June 2012;38(4):501-5.

7. de Jong AEE, Bremer M, Hofland HWC, Schuurmans MJ, Middelkoop E, van Loey NEE. The visual analogue thermometer and the graphic numeric rating scale: A comparison of self-report instruments for pain measurement in adults with burns. Burns. March 1, 2015;41(2):333-40.

8. Van Der Wal MBA, Verhaegen PDHM, Middelkoop E, Van Zuijlen PPM. A Clinimetric Overview of Scar Assessment Scales: J Burn Care Res. 2012;33(2):e79-87.

9. Draaijers LJ, Tempelman FRH, Botman YAM, Kreis RW, Middelkoop E, van Zuijlen PPM. Colour evaluation in scars: tristimulus colorimeter, narrow-band simple reflectance meter or subjective evaluation? Burns J Int Soc Burn Inj. March 2004;30(2):103-7.

10. Draaijers LJ, Botman YAM, Tempelman FRH, Kreis RW, Middelkoop E, Van Zuijlen PPM. Skin elasticity meter or subjective evaluation in scars: a reliability assessment. Burns. March 2004;30(2):109-14.

11. Pietrzak WS, Eppley BL. Platelet Rich Plasma: Biology and New Technology. J Craniofac Surg. Nov 2005;16(6):1043-54.

12. Picard F, Hersant B, Bosc R, Meningaud J. The growing evidence for the use of platelet-rich plasma on diabetic chronic wounds: A review and a proposal for a new standard care. Wound Repair Regen. Sept 2015;23(5):638-43.

13. Ferrari M, Zia S, Valbonesi M, Henriquet F, Venere G, Spagnolo S, et al. A new technique for hemodilution, preparation of autologous platelet-rich plasma and intraoperative blood salvage in cardiac surgery. Int J Artif Organs. Jan 1987;10(1):47-50.

14. Lubkowska A, Dołęgowska B, Banfi G. Growth factor content in PRP and their applicability in medicine. J Biol Regul Homeost Agents. 2012;26(2 Suppl 1):3S-22S.

15. Kakudo N, Kushida S, Minakata T, Suzuki K, Kusumoto K. Platelet-rich plasma promotes epithelialization and angiogenesis in a splitthickness skin graft donor site. Med Mol Morphol. Dec 2011;44(4):233-6.

16. Miller JD, Rankin TM, Hua NT, Ontiveros T, Giovinco NA, Mills JL, et al. Reduction of pain via platelet-rich plasma in split-thickness skin graft donor sites: a series of matched pairs. Diabet Foot Ankle. 22 Jan 2015;6:10.3402/dfa.v6.24972.

17. Moojen DJF, Everts PAM, Schure R, Overdevest EP, Van Zundert A, Knape JTA, et al. Antimicrobial activity of platelet-leukocyte gel against *Staphylococcus aureus*. J Orthop Res. March 2008;26(3):404-10.

18. Marck RE, Middelkoop E, Breederveld RS. Considerations on the Use of Platelet-Rich Plasma, Specifically for Burn Treatment: J Burn Care Res. 2014;35(3):219-27.

19. Evers LH, Bhavsar D, Mailänder P. The biology of burn injury. Exp Dermatol. Sept 2010;19(9):777-83.

20. Borzini P, Balbo V, Mazzucco L. Platelet Concentrates for Topical Use: Bedside Device and Blood Transfusion Technology. Quality and Versatility. Curr Pharm Biotechnol. 1 May 2012;13(7):1138-44.

21. Marck RE, Gardien KLM, Stekelenburg CM, Vehmeijer M, Baas D, Tuinebreijer WE, et al. The application of platelet-rich plasma in the treatment of deep dermal burns: A randomized, double-blind, intra-patient controlled study. Wound Repair Regen. Jul 2016;24(4):712-20.

22. Van Der Veer WM, Bloemen MCT, Ulrich MMW, Molema G, Van Zuijlen PP, Middelkoop E, et al. Potential cellular and molecular causes of hypertrophic scar formation. Burns. Feb 2009;35(1):15-29.

23. Kotsovilis S, Markou N, Pepelassi E, Nikolidakis D. The adjunctive use of platelet-rich plasma in the therapy of periodontal intraosseous defects: a systematic review. J Periodontal Res. June 2010;45(3):428-43.

24. Dhurat R, Sukesh MS. Principles and Methods of Preparation of Platelet-Rich Plasma: A Review and Author's Perspective. J Cutan Aesthetic Surg. Dec 2014;7(4):189.

25. Kirwan CC, Byrne GJ, Kumar S, McDowell G. Platelet release of Vascular Endothelial Growth Factor (VEGF) in patients undergoing chemotherapy for breast cancer. J Angiogenesis Res. 24 Oct 2009;1:7.

26. Shen E, Chou T, Gau C, Tu H, Chen Y, Fu E. Releasing growth factors from activated human platelets after chitosan stimulation: a possible bio-material for platelet-rich plasma preparation. Clin Oral Implants Res. Oct 2006;17(5):572-8.

27. Yeung CY, Hsieh PS, Wei LG, Hsia LC, Dai LG, Fu KY, et al. Efficacy of Lyophilised Platelet-Rich Plasma Powder on Healing Rate in Patients With Deep Second Degree Burn Injury: A Prospective Double-Blind Randomized Clinical Trial. Ann Plast Surg. Feb 2018;80(2S):S66-9.

28. Prochazka V, Klosova H, Stetinsky J, Gumulec J, Vitkova K, Salounova D, et al. Addition of platelet concentrate to Dermo-Epidermal Skin Graft in deep burn trauma reduces scarring and need for revision surgeries. Biomed Pap Med Fac Univ Palacky Olomouc Czechoslov. 27 Sep 2013;158(2):242.

29. Picard F, Hersant B, Bosc R, Meningaud J. Should we use platelet-rich plasma as an adjunct therapy to treat "acute wounds," "burns," and "laser therapies": A review and a proposal of a quality criteria checklist for further studies. Wound Repair Regen. March 2015;23(2):163-70.

30. Shan GQ, Zhang YN, Ma J, Li YH, Zuo DM, Qiu J lang, et al. Evaluation of the Effects of Homologous Platelet Gel on Healing Lower Extremity Wounds in Patients With Diabetes. Int J Low Extrem Wounds. March 2013;12(1):22-9.

31. Saffle JR. Closure of the Excised Burn Wound: Temporary Skin Substitutes. Clin Plast Surg. Oct 2009;36(4):627-41.

32. Barker CF, Markmann JF. Historical Overview of Transplantation. Cold Spring Harb Perspect Med. Apr 2013;3(4):a014977.

33. Moscona A, Moscona H. The dissociation and aggregation of cells from organ rudiments of the early chick embryo. J Anat. 1952;86:287-301.

34. Sabeh G, Sabé M, Ishak S, Sweid R. New procedure: do sequential skin cell grafts heal third-degree burns? A comparative study of 517 patients. Ann Burns Fire Disasters. 30 Sep 2018;31(3):213.

35. Gimble JM, Katz AJ, Bunnell BA. Adipose-Derived Stem Cells for Regenerative Medicine. Circ Res. May 11, 2007;100(9):1249.

36. Kim WS, Park BS, Kim HK, Park JS, Kim KJ, Choi JS, et al. Evidence supporting antioxidant action of adipose-derived stem cells: Protection of human dermal fibroblasts from oxidative stress. J Dermatol Sci. Feb 2008;49(2):133-42.

37. Werner S, Krieg T, Smola H. Keratinocyte-Fibroblast Interactions in Wound Healing. J Invest Dermatol. May 2007;127(5):998-1008.

38. Grasset N, Raffoul W, Bigliardi P. Bioactive dressings. Rev Med Suisse. 2010;6:354-7.

39. Stenman S, Vaheri A. Distribution of a major connective tissue protein, fibronectin, in normal human tissues. J Exp Med. 1 Apr 1978;147(4):1054-64.

40. Owen RW, Giacosa A, Hull WE, Haubner R, Würtele G, Spiegelhalder B, et al. Olive-oil consumption and health: the possible role of antioxidants. Lancet Oncol. Oct 2000;1(2):107-12.

41. Molan PC. The role of honey in the management of wounds. J Wound Care. Sept 1999;8(8):415-8.

42. White JW, Subers MH, Schepartz AI. THE IDENTIFICATION OF INHIBIN, THE ANTIBACTERIAL FACTOR IN HONEY, AS HYDROGEN PEROXIDE AND ITS ORIGIN IN A HONEY GLUCOSE-OXIDASE SYSTEM. Biochim Biophys Acta. 1963;

43. Beckman MJ, Shields KJ, Diegelmann RF. Collagen metabolism. Wounds: a compendium of clinical research and practice. 2001 Sep;13:177-82.

44. Clouse LH, Comp PC. The regulation of hemostasis: the protein C system. N Engl J Med. 1986 May 15;314(20):1298-304.

45. Salles AG, Gemperli R, Toledo PN, Ferreira MC. Combined Tretinoin and Glycolic Acid Treatment Improves Mouth Opening for Postburn Patients. Aesthetic Plast Surg. June 2006;30(3):356-62.

46. Mecott GA, Al-Mousawi AM, Gauglitz GG, Herndon DN, Jeschke MG. The Role of Hyperglycemia in Burned Patients: Evidence-Based Studies. Shock Augusta Ga. Jan 2010;33(1):10.1097/SHK.0b013e3181af0494.

47. Cunningham-Rundles S, McNeeley DF, Moon A. Mechanisms of nutrient modulation of the immune response. J Allergy Clin Immunol. June 2005;115(6):1119-28.

48. Block J, Hetherington. Facial fat grafting with a prototype injection control device. Clin Cosmet Investig Dermatol. Sep 2013;201.

49. Coleman SR. Hand rejuvenation with structural fat grafting. Plast Reconstr Surg. 2002 Dec;110(7):1731-44.

50. Coleman SR. Structural fat grafting: more than a permanent filler. Plast Reconstr Surg. 2006 Sep;118(3 Suppl):108S-120S

51. Condé-Green A, Baptista LS, Gontijo de Amorin NF, de Oliveira ED, Ribeiro da Silva K, da Silva Gouveia Pedrosa C, et al. Effects of centrifugation on cell composition and viability of aspirated adipose tissue processed for transplantation. Aesthet Surg J. 2010;30(2):249-55.

52. Zuk PA, Zhu M, Ashjian P, De Ugarte DA, Huang JI, Mizuno H, et al. Human adipose tissue is a source of multipotent stem cells. Mol Biol Cell. 2002 Dec;13:4279-95.

53. Li P, Guo X. A review: therapeutic potential of adipose-derived stem cells in cutaneous wound healing and regeneration. Stem Cell Res Ther. 8 Nov 2018;9:302.

54. Trottier V, Marceau-Fortier G, Germain L, Vincent C, Fradette J. IFATS collection: using human adipose-derived stem/stromal cells for the production of new skin substitutes. Stem Cells. 2008 Oct;26(10):2713-23

55. Noszczyk B, Krześniak N. Fat grafts in the reconstruction and treatment of chronic wounds. Pol J Surg. 2013 Dec;85(12):937-41

56. Piccolo NS, Piccolo MS, Piccolo MT. Fat grafting for treatment of burns, burn scars, and other difficult wounds. Clin Plast Surg. 2015;42:263-83

57. Abouzaid AM, El Mokadem ME, Aboubakr AK, Kassem MA, Al Shora AK, Solaiman A. Effect of autologous fat transfer in acute burn wound management: A randomized controlled study. Burns. Sept 2022;48(6):1368-85.

58. Klinger M, Marazzi M, Vigo D, Torre M. Fat injection for cases of severe burn outcomes: a new perspective of scar remodeling and reduction. Aesth Plast Surg. 2008;32:465-9.

59. Fredman R, Katz AJ, Hultman CS. Fat grafting for burn, traumatic, and surgical scars. Clin Plast Surg. 2017 Oct;44(4):781-91.

APPENDIX

The steps in the sequential skin cell grafting procedure (34) are as follows:

Step 1: Preparing the areas to be treated

This first stage consists of treating the burns according to standard procedures: debridement, cleaning and application of dressings (silver sulphaguanidine or honey). Contaminated or necrotic tissue must be excised within 2 to 4 days for superficial burns (IIP) and 3 to 7 days for deep burns (III).

Step 2: Application of grafts

Allografts or xenografts are used temporarily to protect clean wounds before the application of GSCCs.

Step 3: Sampling healthy skin

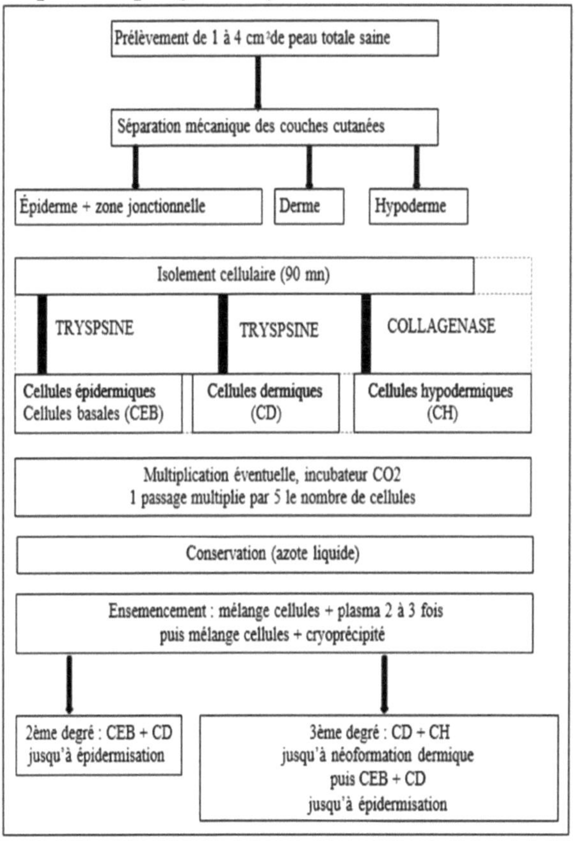

Prélèvement de 1 à 4 cm²de peau totale saine

Séparation mécanique des couches cutanées

Épiderme + zone jonctionnelle | Derme | Hypoderme

Isolement cellulaire (90 mn)

TRYSPSINE | TRYSPSINE | COLLAGENASE

Cellules épidermiques Cellules basales (CEB) | **Cellules dermiques** (CD) | **Cellules hypodermiques** (CH)

Multiplication éventuelle, incubateur CO2
1 passage multiplie par 5 le nombre de cellules

Conservation (azote liquide)

Ensemencement : mélange cellules + plasma 2 à 3 fois
puis mélange cellules + cryoprécipité

2ème degré : CEB + CD
jusqu'à épidermisation

3ème degré : CD + CH
jusqu'à néoformation dermique
puis CEB + CD
jusqu'à épidermisation

Take an elliptical area of healthy skin (1 to 4 cm long and 1 cm wide) from a hairy area, including the epidermis and the superficial dermal junction. The dermis and hypodermis are then separated and sent to the laboratory for preparation.

Stage 4: Cell transformation and use of suspensions
The cells are isolated by enzymatic hydrolysis (trypsin for the epidermal and dermal layers, collagenase for the hypodermis). The suspensions, containing 6 to 7 million cells/cm², are applied to the wounds. The first inoculations use a GSCC/PRP mixture, followed by the addition of plasma cryoprecipitate (CP) from the 3rd or 4th inoculation. Complete coverage is checked with a vital stain (methylene blue).

The cells to be seeded are chosen according to the depth of the burn:

- For superficial burns (IIP): A mixture of epidermo-junctional and dermal cells is applied. The wound goes through a fibrination phase (whitish) followed by a budding phase (reddish) with desquamation. The crusts gradually fall off, giving way to skin that regains its normal colour and sensitivity.
- For deep burns (III): Treatment begins by seeding dermal and hypodermal cells to rebuild dermal tissue, forming bridges and filling in lesions. Next, a mixture of epidermal-junctional and dermal cells is applied to create a new epidermis, with the skin taking on a pale pink hue and areas of epidermis appearing in the centre and around the edges.

Summary

Issue: Burns are a major public health issue, with considerable repercussions on patients' quality of life. Although traditional methods of healing have long prevailed, they can be hampered by various factors such as infection, graft rejection and the risk of hypertrophic or keloid scars. Regenerative therapy is emerging as a promising alternative for the treatment of acute burns, although its integration into clinical practice is controversial due to variable results and ethical challenges, making its considered use essential.

Aim of the work: The aim is to review recent studies on the application of regenerative therapy for the healing of acute burns. This review synthesises emerging innovations, assesses their reliability and safety, and explores challenges and future prospects.

Methods: This was a systematic review based on a comprehensive search of relevant databases, including PubMed, Science Direct and ResearchGate, covering the publication period 2015 to 2024. Four randomised clinical trials were reviewed, involving platelet-rich plasma (PRP), lyophilised PRP (LRP), sequential skin cell transplantation (SSCT) and autologous fat transfer for the treatment of acute burns.

Results: Results on liquid PRP are heterogeneous. Some studies show an improvement in clinical outcomes such as faster healing and pain relief, while other research shows no significant benefits. This disparity may be explained by the variability of preparation techniques, highlighting the need to standardise PRP preparation and application protocols in order to optimise its efficacy and safety. Freeze-dried PRP has been shown to be effective in the treatment of deep second-degree burns by accelerating healing and reducing bacterial contamination. It offers improved thermal stability, prolonged shelf-life, reduced risk of contamination, and prolonged release of growth factors, reinforcing its regenerative effects. Its ease of storage and administration in the clinic make it even more practical. Sequential skin grafts are a promising alternative for treating severe burns. Effective for deep second-degree burns, they could also benefit third-degree cases, particularly in combination with PRP and cryoprecipitated plasma. These grafts complement other techniques and are particularly useful where there is a shortage of skin or where therapeutic options are limited. Autologous grafting of fat offers significant clinical benefits, in particular by reducing the length of hospital stay, the need for additional surgery and the risk of contractures. In addition, this technique reduces the need for skin grafts and improves scar quality compared with traditional methods.

Conclusion: Although regenerative therapies hold promise for the healing of acute burns, further research is required. Future studies should focus on standardising PRP products, comparing liquid and freeze-dried PRP, optimising application protocols, and evaluating sequential and autologous fat skin grafts. These efforts will improve clinical outcomes and the management of acute burns

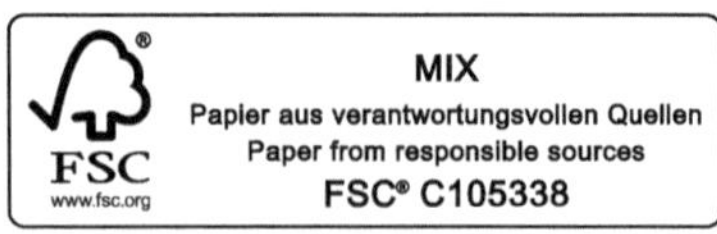

Printed by Books on Demand GmbH, Norderstedt / Germany